I0411377

# FIFTY GREAT WEIGHT LOSS TIPS

**All Rights Reserved © 2013 David Sadtler**

# Contents

# PREFACE

During much of my adult life, I had been overweight. Never obese, but overweight. But I could not overlook the overwhelming evidence about the negative health implications of weighing too much. Since I have been an enthusiastic walker and runner for many years, I wanted to be able to continue these pursuits as I got older. So does my wife Mary. Thus our growing interest in weight and nutrition.

I must at this point address one contentious issue, that of whether obese and overweight people can justifiably claim that their weight is not their fault. The growing science of brain function and its relationship to the feeling of fullness is demonstrating that some people don't get this signal effectively and in a timely way. Thus they keep eating beyond the point where they should stop. Several of my hints address this timing problem. Drug companies are addressing this mechanism and much is being written about it. My position is this. You still have to take off the weight or you will have to accept the terrifying consequences of health failure and all of the other undesirable results of being too heavy (see Tips 35, 36, 37, and 38). I sympathise, but it changes nothing.

If you are serious about losing weight, you really have to do five things. Most importantly, you have to eat the right things. Weight loss is hopeless without this. Second, you must moderate how much you eat. Third, you must manage your environmental influences. Unless you're a hermit, there are plenty of weight-related influences around you and you must be aware of them. Fourth, you must tend to your own attitude and outlook and the way in which this will influence the success of weight loss. And finally, you must get exercise. These five requirements are the basis of the fifty great weight loss tips which follow.

A friend asked me if I would identify just the four or five tips that are essential, the most powerful, the ones that would really make a difference. Okay. I think they are these. Banish sugar (Tip 1), weigh yourself each morning (Tip 15), eat slowly (Tip 16), consider the impact on your health (Tip 35), and commit or forget it (Tip 43). You might pick others.

One more thing. This short book is not for the faint-hearted. It has been written in a direct and unapologetically tough way. We all have to be tough about defeating overweight and obesity. It is a grave threat to mankind.

Now, here are the tips.

# MANAGING WHAT YOU EAT

It couldn't be simpler. In order to take off weight and keep it off, you must confine yourself to eating the right foods and you must reject the wrong ones. If you like donuts and refuse to give them up, read no further, since you are not going to make it. But if you are willing to consider what is healthy and appropriate for good nutrition and weight control, read on.

# Tip 1 – Banish Sugar

If I was limited to offering only one tip for losing weight, it would be to banish sugar.

All forms of sugar - sucrose, the white stuff in the bowl, fructose, the sugar in fruit, and some amazingly insidious stuff called high fructose corn syrup - will make you fat. And cutting it out will have a quick and discernible effect on your waistline. The same goes for honey, molasses, maple syrup, and so on.

Get used to drinking your coffee and tea without sugar. Just that will have a visible impact if you drink a lot of these drinks and with sugar - especially if you have two or three teaspoonfuls. Just stop. I did it some years ago. It wasn't that bad. Really.

Next stop all fizzy drinks. They are loaded with sugar. Don't even drink fruit juice (see Tip 3), because they add sugar to that too. Even if it says "no sugar added", it still contains the natural sugar, fructose. You can reduce the harmful impact of fructose in fruit by eating the fruit itself because the fibre you ingest along with it processes the sugar in a better way. But forget fruit juice.

You must also look out for sugar in packaged and processed foods. Read the labels. See if there is any sugar in the product. You'll be amazed. Manufacturers put sugar in nearly everything. Notable examples are ketchup, baked beans, breakfast cereals, yoghurts, and on and on. We use sugar-free muesli. All the major supermarkets stock a private label version. Virtually every other cereal has sugar. Pass it by. Read the labels!

Much current discussion, including advocacy by New York's Mayor Mike Bloomberg, addresses the possibility of the labelling of added sugar. Unsurprisingly, the food industry is fighting this possible development fiercely. The US Department of Agriculture estimates that the average American consumes an incredible 32 teaspoons of added sugar per day in its food. No wonder there is a national obesity crisis!

Mostly in America, but also in the UK, something called high fructose corn syrup or just fructose syrup is added as a cheap sugar substitute. The destructive effect of this stuff has finally been discovered in America, where some products now go so far as to advertise that they don't use it.

Sugar not only goes right to your waistline but at high levels of consumption can overwhelm your pancreas as it desperately tries to produce the insulin to deal with today's fantastic levels of sugar consumption. It often gives up, and then - guess what - diabetes! You don't want diabetes (see Tip 35). It can lead to coronary heat disease, blindness, and the need to amputate legs. I'm not kidding.

Some websites will advise you that sugar is OK as "part of a balanced diet". Don't believe it. They are supporting a large industry that wants to maintain its consumer franchise. And forget looking for help from most politicians, other than Mike Bloomberg, who are afraid of losing the money from and employment in these industries.

BANISH SUGAR!

## Tip 2 – Go easy on stevia

There is a miracle product called Stevia, which people with an uncontrollable sweet tooth swear by. It's a South American herb, something called Stevia rebaudiana. It is held by many in the weight loss forums which I study to be an answer to their sugar addiction. It doesn't take much to satisfy their sweet craving, since it is many times sweeter than sugar and is alleged to have no health risks. It has been used for decades in Japan with no apparent health risks. No problem then. Right?

No. Here is the problem. Not only is sugar the enemy, but the craving for it is what is killing people. The addictive sweet tooth is a malign influence in our bodies. It is what drives the excessive consumption of fizzy drinks and the like. Using Stevia simply perpetuates this addiction. It is like saying, I cannot control my craving for sugar, so I am going to find a way to live with it.

Please note that this tip tells you to go easy on Stevia and does not forbid it. If you simply cannot live without the sweet taste, use it. At least it won't kill you. On the other hand, make sure that you avoid all other forms of sugar. Don't let down your guard. And try to reduce your dependence on it by gradually reducing your use of it (see Tip 20).

# Tip 3 – Don't drink fruit juice

I admit that the command not to drink fruit juice sounds extreme, if not counterintuitive. After all, do we not think of fruit juice as a lovely, natural, healthy drink? But there are good reasons for my condemnation.

Most importantly, as I pointed out in the first tip, fruit juices contain sugar, the bane of all dieters. For the avoidance of doubt, let me once again repeat: sugar is the enemy! You must go all the way in eliminating it from your diet. Not only will this help you to lose weight but it will also make it far less likely that you will contract diabetes. Let us not mince words. Diabetes is a dread disease, one that can result in blindness, heart trouble, and amputated limbs.

Fruit juice is highly likely to have sugar added to it to make it taste even sweeter. Most of the fruit juice in my local Tesco has sugar added to it. I have looked. The sugar added fruit juices are unhealthy in the extreme.

Even if sugar has not been added, even if the label says no sugar added, you should still avoid it. This is because all fruit contains fructose, which is simply another form of sugar. Incredibly most fruit juices with no sugar added actually contain more sugar in the form of fructose than a can of Coca-Cola.

But if you take your fructose in the form of the fruit from which it came, the fibre in the fruit will help protect you somewhat from the fattening effects of the sugar. The fibre leads to some sort of complicated chemical process that makes it less likely that it will be absorbed by your system. Therefore, it is okay to eat a modest amount of fruit every day. It is not okay to ingest it in the form of juice.

Don't drink it.

# Tip 4 – Beware of treats

You may not like this one.

A frequent piece of advice to you dieters is to give yourself the occasional treat – the odd doughnut, scoop of ice cream, piece of Black Forest gateau, etc. After all, you've worked hard, you've accomplished some success, and you deserve a reward. Just a little bit can't hurt.

I think it can, I'm against it, and here is why.

The key to successful dieting, the sina qua non, is total commitment. I have more to say about commitment in Tip 43. You must talk yourself into the idea that you will succeed and achieve your goal – permanent weight loss reduction – no matter what. It can't be casual. You can't say well, I'll give it a try and see if it works. The reason that 95% of diets fail is that the necessary commitment is lacking. Lapsing eventually sets in. The key is a commitment to a life-changing rejection of bad life style habits.

Eating the kind of stuff that one consumes as a treat is simply an extension of one of these habits – eating awful stuff that makes you fat. Calling something a treat enshrines it as something good, something desirable. No it isn't. It's destructive. You should look at a doughnut as the enemy, not a long lost friend. Believe that.

Of course you might identify raw carrots as a treat. I do. Obviously OK. What I'm arguing against is bad treats. You know what I mean.

NO BAD TREATS!

## Tip 5 – Eat more fiber/fibre

The F plan diet was a best-selling book in the 1980s by fellow Canterbury resident Audrey Eyton. Her premise was simple. Making sure that there is a lot of fibre in your diet aids digestion and helps prevent absorption of fat content into the body's cells. The greater bulk of what is eaten also deters overeating by signalling a full stomach sooner. A high-fibre diet also helps prevent constipation.

High-fibre foods include avocados, bran, broccoli, green peas, lentils, oats, raspberries, brown rice, and soya beans. If you want a longer list and the fibre content in such foods, simply Google high fibre foods and you will get plenty of lists. And if you really want to get into this, find yourself a used copy – it is out of print now – of Audrey's book. It sold several million just in the UK in the 1980s, so the message was certainly taken to heart then.

It works.

## Tip 6 – Drink green tea

For information, green tea comes from a specific tea plant: Camellia sinensis. But it is processed quite differently from black tea with no fermentation and less drying. In this way nutrients that are good for your health are better preserved.

There are two reasons you should drink green tea if you want to lose weight.

First, they have discovered a powerful ingredient, EGCG, a powerful anti-oxidant, in green tea. It is being shown to reduce the incidence of certain cancers, and a number of other scary diseases. It also has a big effect on cholesterol levels and helps to fight obesity. It is quite a technical matter, so Google EGCG+obesity if you want to get up to speed.

A second creative use is as a line of demarcation. A blogger put me on to this. After his final meal of the day, he has a cup of green tea. He has decided that that this cup is a line of demarcation which constitutes the end of eating for the day. Some people brush their teeth right after the final meal for the same reason. You are saying to yourself, OK that's it for the day; no more food.

Don't gorge yourself on it though. It contains caffeine and It will keep you awake if you drink too much and too late in the day.

Mary's acupuncturist says, as she leaves, not goodbye or see you later but – DRINK GREEN TEA!

# Tip 7 – Consider vegetarianism

This is a tricky one, not least because there are social, cultural, and ethical forces and attitudes at work when considering vegetarianism.

This subject - whether vegetarianism leads to weight loss - has been exhaustively examined. What is undeniable is that there is considerably less obesity among vegetarians since they typically consume fewer calories than non-vegetarians . The dietary benefit of being a vegetarian lies in the fact that one is directed more toward the kinds of food that everyone should eat more of, fruits, vegetables, fibre-rich foods, and so forth, but the benefits can be undone by not giving up on high-fat products like cheese, butter, and other fatty foods and by not cutting back sufficiently on sugar.

Vegetarians consume fewer calories. That alone explains why they are less obese. But why is this? My guess is that anyone who embarks on this regime has actually given some thought to diet, nutrition, and lifestyle choices. Such people tend to think for themselves and take responsibility for their health. This fact alone separates them out from the vast majority of the population, and in particular from most of the obese. You may not like hearing this but that is what I think and believe.

Another option is to go part way and become a flexitarian. That's what we do. Our diet is highly concentrated on fruit and vegetables high-fibre foods and fish. But we still have the occasional steak from the excellent butcher around the corner. We just don't make a habit of it.

One word of warning here. Several vegetarians I know also avoid dairy products. This may be for ideological reasons in that they want to be nice to the cow. There are also some reasonable nutritional arguments against dairy products. But this is a weight loss book. The problem is that a lack of calcium, which dairy products provide, seems to inhibit the body's ability to burn up fat and calcium supplements don't help much. I am not sure how bulletproof the science is but it sounds plausible, so be careful with this one.

The bottom line is this: vegetarianism is not a foolproof weight loss program in itself but it can lead you in the right direction.

## Tip 8 – Maintain stocks of fast healthy food

Keep an ample supply of tasty healthy snacks on hand, the domestic version of fast food. Try having cut up raw carrots, prewashed vegetables, whole-grain crackers, almonds, and the like. The idea is to compose a list of healthy, low-calorie, low-fat food which you like and which is convenient for a quick snack. You might even include microwave popcorn, tins of chopped tomatoes which can be warmed up, pre-cooked grilled chicken breasts, and the like. Compile your own list and try different things. Just be sure of their nutritional value.

And what about dried fruit? They make great snacks. But, on a recent visit to the supermarket, I was instructed to buy dried apricots and dried prunes. I looked at the ingredients and was stunned to notice that each of these products was about one third sugar. In some packs I find it actually over 50%! A disaster. The reason you like this stuff is because it is very sweet. Forget it.

Fast healthy food means just that. Good nutritionally and low in calories.

## Tip 9 – Clean out your food shelves

This one might be tough.

By now, you must have a pretty good idea of what kind of food is healthy and what isn't. If you are really honest, you know what kind of food is bad and should not be in your house.

So here it is. Go through your refrigerator and your shelves to identify all the bad stuff and throw it out. Don't even give it to the well-intentioned food collections for starving people because you will just be making them unhealthy as well.

And don't make the mistake, ludicrous as it sounds, made by one of our friends. He finally agreed that he had to get rid of the chocolate in the house. His solution was to find it all and eat it all so that there would not be any left. Words fail me.

Do it. No treats.

## Tip 10 – Beware of reliance on low fat products

This tip may sound risky, but the problem lies in over reliance on low fat content as a key to successful weight reduction. I know this to be true, as I made the same mistake myself.

There is some relevant history here. Professor Robert Lustig at the University of California at San Francisco explained it in a famous YouTube video. The concern about obesity in the US in the 1970s led to a major low-fat initiative on the part of food processors, and it was a big commercial success. But epidemiologists noted that the levels of obesity continued to increase despite this major shift to lower fat in packaged foods. The problem was that the lowering of fat made many foods less palatable, a problem which was solved by the introduction of something called high fructose corn syrup. The fat may have been lower, but the calories were shooting up and obesity levels continued to increase. Low fat by itself isn't good enough.

Similarly, don't load up your plate with multiple helpings just because lower fat content is promised.

Of course it is a good idea to reduce the fat content of what you eat. But don't ignore calories and in particular any form of added sugar.

# Tip 11 – Don't ruin healthy food

We all know that salads are healthy. Fresh fruits and vegetables of all kinds are good for you and we should all be sure that we eat substantial amounts.

But the benefit will be greatly reduced if we then drench the salad with high calorie dressing of different kinds. Fast food restaurants are particularly adept at this trick. They sell you a salad which looks really healthy and then cover it with sauce loaded with sugar and high-fat ingredients. Mary's policy on this is to ask for her dressing on the side. She can then drizzle a tiny quantity on the salad and then complete the process with a bit of olive oil and balsamic vinegar, which most restaurants will provide.

Once again, I must admit culpability. I have a weakness for mayonnaise. Ketchup is another dangerous addition. If you don't believe me just look at the ingredients and note the sugar and fat content.

# Tip 12 – Beware of product trickery

Here is how they fool you. The product promotes itself as healthy by touting ingredients like fiber, calcium, and omega-3 fatty acids, which really are good for you. The problem often is that they are also loaded with sugar or salt or something else you really don't want to consume too much of.

I read a letter to the editor of a walking magazine by a lady who had taken up long walks on weekends and was expressing surprise that she was not losing any weight. She reported that all she had to eat when on the trail were granola bars. The truth is that she was gaining more calories from the sugar in the granola bars than she was walking off. But the product was promoted as a healthy, natural food. How could she go wrong? The answer: by not reading the ingredients on the package.

Read the ingredients!

# Tip 13 – Ask the doctor

It might sound obvious that you should talk to your doctor (or nurse or other health care provider) about your weight. But evidence suggests that many doctors don't bother to bring it up. They look at you and maybe figure that it's a waste of time. Or maybe they are fat themselves and are embarrassed to bring up the subject. Or they are afraid of offending you. Or they don't want to get beaten up. Whatever the reason, the record is not good.

You should bring it up. A number of studies have demonstrated that people who discuss their weight with doctors are more successful at losing it. Of course that may be simply a question of people who have already decided that there is a problem wanting to talk about it.

The value of these discussions is information. Patients discover the tremendous health problems which arise from obesity when told face to face by their doctors and are often more likely to act on it. The dangers are many and frightening (see Tip 35).

## MANAGING HOW MUCH YOU EAT

It stands to reason that the more you eat, the more you will weigh. There are many reasons why we eat more than we should. At its most elemental level, it probably goes back to the days when we were all living in caves and had to load up as best we could in order to survive the winter. There are many ways to address this natural inclination. Here are a few.

# Tip 14 – Stay Out of the Kitchen

Unless you're cooking.

If you eat in the kitchen, consider taking your meals elsewhere. In the dining room, for example, if you have one. That's why they call it a dining room. If you must eat in the kitchen, call that end of the room the dining room. Try and separate - in your mind - your place to eat from your place to store and prepare food.

The problem with the kitchen is that it contains food, over and above what is planned for the meal. That leads to snacking, grazing, and so on. Just walking through the kitchen and seeing food can stimulate cravings you might not otherwise have.

Of course you'll have to be in the kitchen to prepare food. It's a good place to be if you are preparing responsible, nutritious food. But everyone else would be well advised to stay out.

And whatever you do, sit at a table with your feet under it, in a chair, when you eat. Don't eat in front of a television or computer or while doing the wash or painting the kid's room. What you are trying to do is to train yourself to eat only when sitting at the table. If you can convince yourself that that is the only time and way to eat, you have a better chance of eliminating casual snacking.

This diet business is all about getting your head right. You have to be committed. The reason that most diets fail is that the requisite commitment is lacking. So – this is where we eat – no place else!

# Tip 15 – Weigh yourself each morning

This is crucial. You need to track progress, constantly, for several reasons.

First you need to see the results of your efforts. Sometimes it takes a while for the improved habits to show results. We've experienced occasional plateauing – where we reached a level and then didn't' make further progress. Then we moved to a new lower level. You need to track what you are achieving so that you are in command. You are in charge. You are managing this life-enhancing process.

Second you need to figure out what works and what can put on the pounds. When we slip, we will say something like, well that's because we drank too much wine last night or it's the cheese we had with lunch. We pretty much now know what will produce both ups and downs because we weigh ourselves every morning. We have established a tight link between behaviour and results. You must as well.

Further, there is a growing body of discouraging evidence which indicates that the body can itself resist weight loss.

There seems to be some remembered equilibrium point in one's weight which the body attempts to retain. If you go below that weight, the body will somehow try and restore it. That means you have to try all the harder when eliminating the habits of a lifetime. You simply must track this closely if you are to succeed, and this means using the scales every morning.

You will hear people say you shouldn't weigh yourself too often because you might get discouraged. Sorry. That's for wimps. You need to be in charge!

Oh, and get yourself a decent set of scales. Preferably with a digital readout so that there is no room for equivocal interpretation of what the scales tell you. Get a good one. It is a mechanical link to the rest of your life.

# Tip 16 – Eat slowly

This may seem like a trivial point. It isn't. It is a powerful tool in fighting over-eating. I'll keep coming back to it.

It seems that there's a signal that gets passed from your stomach to your brain that says, OK, I'm full, I don't need any more. There is something of a time lag involved – in some people longer than others. But it is usually estimated at about 20 minutes. Much of the search for a good obesity pill addresses this lag and seeks to reduce it.

So the first thing is to realise that there is a lag. Hey, maybe if I slow down a little I won't feel so hungry.

In the Mediterranean countries, they don't manage their finances very well, but they know how to eat. En famille.

Around a table. It's an occasion and it lasts a lot longer than here. They are less obese then we. They just don't eat so fast.

My wife has a relevant saying: "the moment passes". Just wait. Slow down. And you won't eat so much.

# Tip 17 – Respect the numbers

Managing your decisions by looking at the numbers may not be your first instinct. But many dodgy businesses count on the fact that you don't look at the numbers too closely. And many of us, even after having noted the numbers, don't consider their meaning and their implications for our well-being.

For example the interest rates charged by credit cards when you don't clear your balance each month (incidentally, I am told that careful spenders who do pay everything each month are termed "deadbeats" in the industry), and the rates on payday loans, for example, can be astronomic. People taking out floating rate mortgages at favourable rates often fail to consider what happens when interest rates go up. Negative equity and possible foreclosure is what happens. Don't ignore this stuff. Think about it. It's important.

There is a huge role for numbers in dieting. First and foremost, figure out your BMI (if you are not sure how to do that, refer to the Links section) or waist to height ratio and set a weight goal, one that means that you aren't obese – or overweight. Know the relevant numbers – the specific numbers that will enable you to live longer and healthier and in less discomfort.

Second, decide what your maximum calorie intake should be and then measure what you are actually eating. Even McDonalds is helping in this (not very willingly, I suspect) as they the post calorie content of their food. Use these calorie limits as you read the labels of the food you buy.

You cannot afford to ignore the numbers. They are really your friends. Welcome them!

## Tip 18 – Use a smaller plate

Fascinating research has been undertaken on the subject of visual prompts and how our eating is affected by what we see. One study indicates that colour contrast is important. If all the food is the same colour as the plate, you'll eat more because you don't see the contrast. Thus, it might be a good idea to use black plates, unless of course you are, for some reason, eating black food.

Similarly, using a smaller plate makes intrinsic sense. The smaller the plate, the less you can fit on it. Dinner plates have gradually crept up in size in recent years in people's homes and in restaurants. Have you noticed this? Restaurants are merely responding to market requirements, that is, to gluttony.

A thought leader in this area is Brian Wansink, director of Cornell University's Food and Brand Lab. He refers to this subject as mindful eating, the idea that what you see in front of you affects how you eat it.

## Tip 19 – Drink more water

Drinking more water obviously makes sense. If you fill your stomach with water, there is less room in it for anything else.

Since water contains no calories, drinking water will give you a head start on a successful diet program.

Some people don't like water. The trick therefore is to find a way to make it more palatable. Try adding lemon slices or bits of fruit. Teas infused with herbal ingredients can also help.

There are also metabolic implications. Dehydration can cause complicated changes in bodily chemistry and metabolism which have been shown to inhibit weight loss. Simply put, you need water to stay alive, so drinking more water is a no-brainer.

Do it.


# Tip 20 – Cut back gradually

I admit that it is tough to institute and stick to a responsible diet, especially if it means that you have to make substantial changes in the way you eat now. Therefore, do it gradually.

Count your calorie intake over a period of time, say a week or two. There are excellent tools for doing this online. My favorite is caloriecount.about.com. Then resolve to reduce that intake for the next two weeks by a small amount, say 10% or even 5%. Keep shaving a bit at a time and your weight loss will assuredly follow.

The real dynamic here is one of fighting the very powerful forces of habit. We are used to eating in a certain way and a full frontal assault on that way of life may be impossible for most of us. So do it gradually.

# Tip 21 – Eat spicy food

Eating spicy or strongly seasoned food may help in weight loss. Some research suggests that it also inhibits weight gain.

The idea is this. Any eating process that slows you down is beneficial since it makes your brain wait for the fullness signal. For many, spicy food makes you stop and think about what you are eating. That's good.

One theory relates to Capsaicin, the substance in hot peppers that can give you a real jolt. It is strong stuff and is even used for defensive pepper sprays, so you are strongly advised not to take too much of it, unless you grew up with it for reasons of ethnicity and social groups. One idea is that it increases metabolism which in turn inhibits weight gain.

It isn't foolproof for everyone but surely must be worth a try.


# Tip 22 – Try chopsticks

The idea of using chopsticks to lower food consumption is simple. For most of us they are a bit challenging to use and will certainly slow us down. Even if expert, you can't get that much food onto a pair of chopsticks, so bite-size is apt to be reduced. That's good. Again part of the value of using chopsticks is the exploitation of the time delay to the brain.

Try using chopsticks, even for non-Chinese food.


# Tip 23 – Break it up into pieces

This is another "mindful eating" idea, exploiting the notion that what you think you see in front of you affects how you eat it.

What seems to happen is that for pieces of anything weighing the same as a single piece somehow seem like more to your brain and stomach. You thus are slightly more satisfied. Breaking your food up into pieces may also have the beneficial effect of slowing you down.

## Tip 24 – Turn off the TV

Anything which distracts you from the eating process while you are actually eating seems to lead to greater consumption. People who text, talk on the telephone, watch television, or even drive a car while eating have been shown to eat more than if they can confine themselves just to the eating process. This is one of the reasons that we advocate eating properly at a table and not on the run.

Enjoy your meal, then get up and continue whatever you were doing.

## Tip 25 – Have a decent breakfast

It seems counter intuitive, but people who skip breakfast have more trouble losing weight than those who don't. The principal reason seems to be that having an empty stomach at the start of the day when activity begins leads to disproportionate hunger later on and thus excessive consumption.

Of course I am not suggesting that you gorge yourself at breakfast with fried food, sugared cereals, and the like. Good nutrition at breakfast is also necessary, but be sure you actually have breakfast.

# Tip 26 – Don't get quite full.

For some, leaving food on the plate is a repugnant idea. After all, who can afford to waste food and who can justify it when there are many people who don't have enough?

It is still a good idea. One possible benefit is that it may gradually occur to you to take less food in the first place since you are not eating it all. If you can manage to get into this habit, you have taken an important step. You can thus gradually wean yourself away from larger quantities. Second you are likely to get a reward from the stomach to brain time delay factor. Some minutes later you may even say, I didn't even want that final amount. My wife's phrase for this, as I have mentioned before, is that "the moment passes". It's a powerful idea. Anything that slows you down and makes you realize that you really didn't need that last bite is a good thing.

Exploit it.

# Tip 27 – Beware the sight of extra food

I know this from my own experience. If I see food, especially food that I like, I am probably going to eat it.

So the trick is to prevent me from seeing it. Apart from healthy snacks, keep food out of sight. Avoid putting serving dishes of food on the table, since the instinctive reaction is to reach for more and takes seconds. And be very very careful with buffet meals, whether at home, at parties, at weddings, or in restaurants. The temptation is to really load up the plate with all the good stuff that you like.

Out of sight is out of mind. Exploit this.

## Tip 28 – Chew your food thoroughly

My mother always told me to chew my food carefully, advising me to chew each mouthful a lot more times than I thought necessary. I think she was onto something. By the way, she was never fat.

We have long known that digestion improves with careful chewing. Wolfing one's meal down is more apt to lead to indigestion. That's old news.

But there is an additional benefit for weight loss in that it slows you down. Over and over again I have mentioned the value of eating slowly since it exploits the time lag between the fullness feeling and the fact of actual fullness of the stomach.

So, slow down, chew thoroughly, put your fork down between bites, and enjoy the meal.

## MANAGING YOUR OUTSIDE INFLUENCES

We don't live in a vacuum. There are many outside influences which can affect our attitude toward our food. They can be both positive and negative. We should be aware of them and act accordingly.

# Tip 29 – Tell others what you're doing

Once you really decide to go for it – to take on the commitment to behave responsibly by eating less, eating right, and exercising more - let all your friends and family know what you're setting out to do and what you plan to accomplish.

The big benefit from doing this is the self-creation of pressure on you to keep it up. You don't want to look bad or weak or inept in front of your nearest and dearest, do you?

Also, if they are good people who really care about you, they'll urge you on, encourage you, and tell you it's a great idea (unless they too are fat – see Tip 32).

You'll have to give them progress reports – if only to tell them how much you've lost. If you're really brave, you'll tell them how much you weigh and how much you want to weigh. At work, you might even post a PowerPoint graph of weight loss progress.

You might even get them to pledge sponsorship money; they have to pay out to a designated charity when you reach a certain weight. Or how about this – you have to pay them if you fail. That will really put the pressure on you.

Whatever works.

## Tip 30 – Consider joining a group

If you've followed Tip 29 and announced your plan and even got some money promised for your success, you'll want to use all the tools at your disposal to achieve that success.

There is strength in numbers. It's great if you and your spouse or partner can embark on this adventure together. You encourage each other, discuss progress and what seems to work, and decide on the ultimate target weight together. That's what we did.

But if you don't have that benefit – either because you don't have a significant other or because he or she won't support you (alas often the case – especially if obese him or herself), then you would be well advised to find an external support group.

Furthermore there is evidence that it works. A study at the University of Birmingham (here in the UK) indicates that groups like Weight Watchers have far greater success in inducing weight loss than do "doctor-led" programs. Makes sense to me. One needs constant peer group encouragement and support to make permanent changes.

## Tip 31 – Move to the big city

Moving to a big city to take off weight sounds like a crazy idea, but it isn't. People who live in big cities simply walk around more. They do not get into their cars every time they want to go somewhere. Moving to the city really means getting more exercise.

I admit that doing something like this is quite a radical step as an enabler of weight loss, but, for many of you, this is a life or death struggle.

Consider it.

# Tip 32 – Decide whom to hang out with

OK, this is a tough, maybe brutal idea, but we're about losing weight to save lives, not to pussyfoot around defensive sensibilities.

There is strong evidence that you are more likely to gain weight if you're friends are overweight. Similarly, obese people with slim friends have more success losing weight. A substantial piece of research was done a few years ago with high school students which strongly confirmed this conclusion.

Why might this be? It is probably as simple as this. If you are fat and look around and all of your friends are fat, you won't feel unusual or embarrassed about your weight. You are simply part of the crowd. No problem. But if your friends are a lot slimmer than you, you may be more inclined to respond to peer group pressure and go on a diet.

I know, I know. This is tough love and perhaps hard to take. How could anyone desert one's friends for such a self-centered objective?

The answer is, unfortunately, you have to decide which is more important. As I have said so many times in these tips, successful and permanent weight loss requires total commitment and doing everything possible to achieve the end. This could be one of them.

## Tip 33 – Forget the fads and gimmicks

As if you hadn't noticed, there is an unending stream of new diets, supplements, pills, new age rituals, and the like. All promise a unique answer to the overweight. It goes on and on. There's a lot of money it. As the American circus promoter, PT Barnum, famously said, "there's one born every minute". He meant suckers. Don't be one.

At the end of the day, it's all about what and how much you eat and whether you burn off any of those calories with exercise.

Face the facts. Eat less, eat right, and exercise more. If you are grabbing onto every fad and quack remedy as it comes along, you are kidding yourself. There is no dietary free lunch.

Eat less, eat right, and exercise more.

## Tip 34 – Avoid eating late at night

We try to eat our main meal as early as possible and never late in the evening, unless there is no choice. We sing in a choral society (in Canterbury Cathedral) and usually have a restaurant meal after our concerts to restore energy. Singing a major oratorio is quite tiring. We always gain a pound or two when we have that late meal. But that's only five times a year.

The reason is elusive, some ascribing it to an interaction between sleep, hormones, circadian rhythms, and the like. Some say there is no late night eating penalty at all. It is a long-running and inconclusive debate. Google it and see.

All I know is that we definitely see the penalty. Try it yourself. Resolve not to eat after 6PM for a month and see what happens!

## MANAGING YOUR ATTITUDE

I keep saying that the only way to achieve permanent weight loss is to be obsessively committed to this goal. As in so many areas of human endeavour, the most important ingredient for success is focusing your brain on the task at hand – getting your head right. To do so is half the battle and a great enabler.

# Tip 35 – Consider the impact on your health

Here is a powerful inducement to get serious about weight loss. The fact is that, if you are obese or even overweight, you are likely to die sooner and experience more illness. For many, the experience of retirement is made miserable because of the awful health problems associated with overweight and obesity. Here are the facts.

The five biggest killer diseases in the UK – and it is largely the same in the US - are, in order, coronary heart disease, stroke, infectious disease – which in both the UK and the US means pneumonia and flu - cancer, and diabetes (and its complications). The bad news is that obesity is implicated in all of them.

Not only are you more likely to die sooner when you are obese, but these diseases are very unpleasant to experience. Your quality of life suffers. Coronary heart disease is scary and painful and it prevents you from doing a lot of things you'd like to do, especially active things. Stroke is horrible: you are likely to experience memory loss, incontinence, and speech problems and you can wind up drooling in a chair. The infectious diseases are not only unpleasant in themselves but you can give them to others. Cancer, almost all varieties of which are made more likely by obesity, can be excruciating. And diabetes almost doesn't bear thinking about – unless you don't mind angina, amputated limbs, and blindness.

And if dying sooner and being sick isn't enough of an incentive, how about this? Current research is now demonstrating a link between dementia and obesity. Few things are scarier than the idea of losing one's mind. We are now learning that there is some kind of metabolic link between obesity and brain function and the results are harrowing. I don't want to suffer from senior dementia and neither should you.

Think about this – very seriously and honestly.

## Tip 36 – Consider the impact on the healthcare system

If you have any doubt about the implications of an unhealthy lifestyle, consider what a nurse friend told me not long ago. She said that the wards in the hospital in which she works were filled, nearly exclusively, with people who are obese, get no exercise, don't eat properly and who smoke. There is little question that obesity is imposing an increasingly intolerable burden on the National Health Service. I have already noted the estimate that just treating diabetes takes about 10% of the total budget.

If this were not bad enough, and it is really bad, obese patients injure hospital staff. My wife is a retired nurse and she says that she does not know a career nurse whose back has not been injured by lifting obese patients. How can you not be ashamed when you realize that your bulk is injuring those who care for you?

Think carefully about what you are doing to the healthcare system, wherever you live.

## Tip 37 – Consider the discomfort of others

Overweight and obese people cause difficulty and resentment on airplanes. Many airlines now require passengers above a certain weight or girth to buy an extra seat, an expensive proposition. Passengers of normal weight sitting next to obese passengers often bitterly resent being encroached upon. Some make a real fuss and show indignation and even bitterness. Surely you do not want to be the cause of this.

Obese people are more likely to snore. This keeps others awake. It can not only cause anger and resentment but can even damage marriages.

Obese people are much more apt to smell bad. Bacteria form under layers of fat. This is unpleasant for those around them. I myself had the experience of sitting next to an obese passenger who smelled bad on a long plane flight. I went to a different part of the aircraft, actually abandoning the luxury and comfort for which my company had paid. I really resented that.

Think of other people, not just yourself.

## Tip 38 – Consider what overweight or obesity is doing to your own self esteem

Self-esteem is vital to human beings. The lack of it causes trouble everywhere in the world where people are looked down upon. It is a basic and nearly indispensable need, certainly a desire. The same is true for the obese, and when it is threatened, it can be sad and even overwhelming.

Many receive public scorn and derogatory remarks even when walking down the street. I've seen it myself. It must be awful to experience such denigration.

Obese people often have problems with sex. They find it difficult to attract sexual partners and, even having done so, trouble with copulating satisfactorily. Who wants this?

Think about your self-image. Would you not want to protect and even strengthen it?

# Tip 39 – Get enough sleep

We need adequate sleep to be healthy and happy. It also turns out that we need it in order to keep our weight under control.

It seems that there are a number of hormones whose levels are affected by sleep. Most notably, leptin, which regulates the fullness feeling from the stomach to the brain, is an essential tool in fighting weight gain. Inadequate sleep lowers the levels of this invaluable substance and makes it more likely that you will gain weight.

If you have trouble getting to sleep, make it your business to learn more about why this is. Diet can play a big role in sleeplessness. Whole grains of different sorts, yoghurt, bananas, and fish have all been shown to enhance sleep.

Conversely, high glycemic index foods (e.g., white bread, potatoes, white rice, baguettes, bagels, corn flakes) inhibit it. This is a subject area that you need to understand.

And don't nap during the day if you have any trouble sleeping at night.

Get enough sleep.

# Tip 40 – Clarify your thinking about losing weight

Think about all the reasons you might want to lose weight. There are a lot of possibilities. You may want to look better, feel better, stay healthier, live longer, get more sex, stop receiving scornful looks when walking down the street, and so forth. Whichever of these applies to you, it is an important psychological step to be clear about it. That way, you can set specific goals that reflect these reasons.

Write them down. Make little signs and attach them to the fridge with a magnet. Reinforce your aspirations.

Don't let yourself forget why you need to lose weight.

# Tip 41 – Visualise your ideal weight

Following the previous tip about clarifying your reasons, try to visualize in your mind's eye how you will look when you have lost that weight. Picture yourself wearing new clothes, clothes that will fit your slimmer figure. When you look in the mirror, try and superimpose the desired image on top of what you are actually seeing.

This is all about changing the way you view yourself and your ability to control what you see.

Imagine and enjoy.

## Tip 42 – Have a "never again" weight

At the same time as deciding your reasons for weight loss and your ideal image of yourself, you can also decide on a weight which you will never again be burdened by. You are convincing yourself that your new life precludes the possibility of ever being again at that weight.

As you succeed in your weight loss program, you can even consider moving your "never again" weight downward. The whole idea here is to decide on what aspect of your life and appearance is unacceptable and then take charge to make sure it doesn't happen.

## Tip 43 – Commit or forget it!

You may not like this tip, but it is one of the two most important in the entire list, the other being the first one, to banish sugar. Commitment is not only important, it is essential. The reason that most diets fail is that the necessary, unalterable commitment is lacking. Too many dieters say things like, well I'll try this one and see if it works.

There are many wonderful stories of major weight loss accomplishment in the various on-line forums on this subject.

Nearly all of them reflect an obsessive and irrevocable determination to take off the weight. What they demonstrate, time and time again, is that nothing less will do.

The sheer determination exhibited by film stars to bulk up for a part and then take it off again exemplifies this level of determination and commitment. Who can forget Robert De Niro bulking up for the part of the overweight boxer in Raging Bull? He put on the weight and then he took it off again. Not easy but possible when determined.

Taking off weight, especially a lot of it, isn't easy. If you think it is or if you are embarking upon this effort casually and without total commitment, you are probably wasting your time and should probably forget it. After all, you will save some money by not having to buy a new wardrobe.

Commit or forget it.

## Tip 44 – Think about denial

We are all familiar with the word denial. It means refusing to accept something which is unpleasant or even unbearable. A classic example is the inability to accept the death of loved ones, even to the point of seeing them or hearing them at odd times of day or night. Freud did a lot of work on denial and postulated that people make use of it to protect themselves and their emotional well-being when experiencing overwhelming conflicts.

It can certainly apply to overweight or obese people. It may apply to you. Most commonly, obese people deny that they weigh too much. That is why health organizations promote the use of various measures like body mass index and waist to height ratio. For such people, the first step is similar to that of an alcoholic, which is to acknowledge the problem.

Acknowledge denial. It may help you make the needed commitment to get healthy.

# Tip 45 – Confront boredom

Why would I raise the subject of boredom? This is a weight loss book.

People often just eat for emotional reasons, not necessarily for nutrition or even to satisfy hunger. Hey, I've got nothing to do so I'll eat. To be blunt, use your imagination and find something better to do than just eat.

We all know that our psychological makeup, our emotional profile, our general well-being, are all huge factors in obesity and in managing it. One could almost go so far as to say that getting your head right is the single most important thing you can do in weight-loss. I have raised the subject before when discussing the necessity to confront denial and the overriding urgency of making an irrevocable commitment to weight loss. It really is all in your head. Confronting boredom for what it is and deciding to deal with it directly as a way of distracting yourself from hunger is a great example of this.

A corollary of boredom and the idea that avoiding thinking about what we are doing is the question of lazy habits. Many people work in office buildings and eat in company cafeterias where the same old stuff is pretty much served every day. We don't really think much about it, we just eat it. It's the path of least resistance. After all we have other things to worry about and there is a lot of demanding work waiting for us back at our desks. The problem is that the stuff they are serving may not be nutritional. It may be fatty, loaded with sugar, and not the sort of stuff you would eat if you were really serious about losing weight. But it's there, it's available, and we just eat it. Wrong. A bad habit.

Get interested in what you are eating. Think about what happens when you swallow that doughnut. It is a fascinating subject if only because your life and your ability to enjoy it depend on it, on making the right choices.

# Tip 46 – Manage your hunger

OK, I admit it. There may be, in some people, a defect in the process whereby the stomach tells the brain that it is full. The source of the problem may be genetic and one that expresses itself through hormonal imbalances, dodgy neurotransmitters, and so forth. I am hedging my language a bit because I find the argument on this topic incomplete and poorly advocated at the moment and beset with political agendas. Those who would defend the obese say that this science proves that they are not responsible for their internal bodily physics and chemistry and that we should lay off the criticism.

Wrong.

The point is that some people experience greater hunger than others and at different stages in the process of eating. Some people are light-skinned and some have dark skin. Some are blonde, some have black hair and some are redheads. Not everyone is alike. And not everyone experiences hunger in the same way.

The challenge thus is to acknowledge hunger and manage it positively, rather than giving into it passively and pathetically. If you are beset by hunger and know you don't need further nutrition, for example, by studying nutritional requirement charts for adults, accept the fact that you are often going to feel hungry when you don't need to eat. That's the point. Persuade yourself that this is the truth.

The next step then is to regard excessive hunger as the enemy. This is something you must defeat. Think about the rewards from the victory. If you can manage to eat less, especially of all the bad stuff I have mentioned in earlier tips, you will begin to lose weight. Every overweight person wants this. You are no exception.

So, get your head around hunger. It can be a deceitful, destructive, nasty enemy. Manage it.

## GETTING ADEQUATE EXERCISE

We need exercise to stay healthy. It enhances cardio-vascular fitness and enables our bodies to operate more efficiently. We want our circulatory system to be be good at delivering oxygen to all those cells. That's what exercise does for systemic health.

It also enables weight loss. Of course it burns up calories. But it also seems to do good things to one's metabolic processes and aids digestion and the achievement of proper weight.

# Tip 47 – Do all three (eat right, eat less and get exercise)

There are three sensible ways to lose weight: eat less, eat right, and exercise more. Of course you can get on-line and buy guaranteed diet pills with God knows what results and after-effects. Or you can let a doctor cut you open and tie a string around your stomach. But I'm talking about sensible solutions.

It is also true that taking any one of these three actions to extreme lengths will take off the weight. You can eat practically nothing and slim down. War-time POW and concentration camps demonstrated that. Or you can eat only raw carrots. That'll do it. And you can start walking, then running, then running long distances, and do it most of the day every day. That'll take a long time, since being obese you'll have to start at a snail's pace. But eventually it'll work too.

There are two problems with going with just one – or even two – of these strategies alone. The motivation to go the extremes noted above is extremely unlikely in someone overweight or obese. The start has to be within the realm of possibility.

Also, doing anything extreme as suggested is likely to be damaging to health. Starvation is not good for the metabolism or, for that matter, the ability to hold a job. Eating only carrots will turn you yellow and probably cause some sort of musculature problem. And exercising alone may result in a heart attack if you push it too hard while still fat.

So do them all, slow and easy. Take some simple steps to eat less, like refusing seconds, taking smaller helpings in the first place, and phasing out snacking. Improve the nutritional menu by, for example, banishing sugar. And start walking a bit at a time, but more each day. Follow the tips.

Moderation, but dedication. That's the ticket.

# Tip 48 – Believe in the benefits of exercise

If you are to be a healthy person with a healthy metabolic profile, you simply must exercise. Just staying at home and starving yourself will not result in a good health outcome. You might even be thinner, but you may well not be healthier.

Many people I have met are desperate to denigrate exercise. Guess why. It is because they are either unable or disinclined to do it. And they are jealous of the fact that I get so much benefit from it.

If you are really obese, you will certainly not be able to run marathons right away. But you can start gradually. Short walks each day at an easy pace, gradually building up to a stronger one, can work wonders.

One argument against exercise is that after a vigorous workout you may feel the need to eat a lot to replenish your store of energy. I must say that that has never been my experience. I usually find that exercise actually dulls appetite a bit. Another argument is that you may feel the need to reward yourself for exercise more than you might otherwise do. All I can say is this: get a life, stop making excuses and coming up with alibis for eating too much.

Believe in exercise. It is sensationally good for you.

## Tip 49 – Walk Your Dog

Walking a dog is exercise and they need a lot of walking, especially if big. We know a couple who acquired a beautiful black lab and then just let him run around by himself in the back garden. That beautiful dog is now fat, listless, and sad looking. Awful.

This subject has been studied extensively. Walking is good exercise and makes a major contribution to weight control.. Also, most enjoy the experience; it is not a chore.

I originally thought of calling this tip "get a dog", but my wife pointed out that some people get dogs, walk them a few times, and then ignore them, a cruel treatment for animals that need exercise. If you plan to get a dog as a result of this tip, remember that it is a commitment for the life of a dog to take him or her out regularly, at least twice a day.

Go for it.

**AND FINALLY**

# Tip 50 – Revisit Tip 1 and avoid sugar

Sugar is a huge problem. Some forms of it are digested in a better way than others, but all are ultimately lethal. Face the fact that it is bad for you and then, gradually if necessary, get off it. Looking for substitutes isn't the answer. The idea is to defeat your craving for it, which will never happen as long as you keep finding new ways to get the sweet taste.

In case you have ever been confused about what they call sugar on packaging, the American Heart Association helpfully provides the following terms often used for added sugar: brown sugar, corn sweetener, corn syrup, fruit juice concentrates, high-fructose corn syrup, honey, invert sugar, malt sugar, molasses, raw sugar, sugar, sugar molecules ending in "ose" (dextrose, fructose, glucose, lactose, maltose, sucrose), and syrup. Food packagers will often look for ways to mislead you.

Fight back and live better and longer.

I hope you have picked up some useful ideas from this short booklet that will help you in your weight loss quest. You'll be glad right away of whatever success you manage to achieve and even more so as you get older. Good luck!

# Useful links

I'll not burden you with sources of scientific information on weight and obesity, even though there are many good ones. What I've listed below are those that will be of practical value as you continue on your personal life saving crusade

http://www.nhs.uk/Tools/Pages/Healthyweightcalculator.aspx. A convenient tool for calculating your BMI to determine whether you are normal, overweight, obese. etc. Mercifully, being a UK site, it will accept input in English or metric terms.

http://caloriecount.about.com/. A very useful site. Information about the calorie content of many foods and a calculator to help you decide how many you consumed yesterday. Also contains accounts, often inspirational, of weight reduction success stories.

http://www.nhs.uk/conditions/obesity/pages/introduction.aspx. A good portal into the NHS view of obesity. It provides a short video featuring people who have addressed the obesity problem.

http://www.nhs.uk/Livewell/loseweight/Pages/Tenminuteworkouts.aspx. A useful list of ideas for short exercise workouts for people who have trouble finding the time.

http://www.nhs.uk/change4life/Pages/change-for-life.aspx. A new program called change4life is explained in an interactive website that helps to tailor a weight reduction program to your circumstances. A useful feature is a local search function that identifies locations near you to offer facilities for physical exercise and the like.

http://www.nhs.uk/Video/Pages/Bobobesity.aspx. An amusing cartoon which explains why a couch potato named Bob is obese (in case there is still any doubt in your mind).

http://newsinhealth.nih.gov/issue/Dec2010/Feature1. From America's top health research organisation, the National Institutes of Health (NIH) here offer useful advice on changing the habits that nurture obesity.

http://www.nhs.uk/Livewell/Goodfood/Pages/food-labelling.aspx. An excellent explanation of how to read food labels in the supermarket so as to avoid taking in more than a target amount of fat, calories, and so forth. An essential tool.

.

# Author

David Sadtler is a career writer, teacher, and management consultant specialising in corporate strategy and finance. He has published a number of books and many articles on these subjects. Although still counselling on various investment projects, he has increasingly focused his concern and attention on social issues, and in particular on obesity, since it is becoming the leading public health problem worldwide.

He has written five articles on this subject:

- Diet Tough Talk: Eliminate Sugar (http://amzn.to/UNnCpH)
- Diet Tough Talk: Only Total Commitment Will Do It (http://amzn.to/UNnWog)
- Diet Tough Talk: Obesity Means More Disease And Earlier Death (http://amzn.to/UNnRAX)
- Diet Tough Talk: Realise The Damage You Are Doing (http://amzn.to/UNo2w5)
- Diet Tough Talk: Eat Less (http://amzn.to/UNnN4e)

There are at least two more coming in this series:

- Diet Tough Talk: You Must Exercise
- Diet Tough Talk: Consider Vegetarianism

There is also an earlier book:

- Help! My Husband Is Obese and I'm afraid He'll Die – how to get him to lose weight (http://amzn.to/UNpkY1) It is directed at partners of obese people who are desperate to get a partner or spouse to lose weight; it suggests strategies for doing so.

He can be contacted at david.sadtler@gmail.com and would welcome your comments.

www.ingramcontent.com/pod-product-compliance
Lightning Source LLC
Chambersburg PA
CBHW070501290526
45790CB00003B/1048